TWO M.
A PHARMACIST ASK,
"ARE YOU GETTING IT 5 TIMES A DAY?"

FRUITS AND VEGETABLES

Enzymes, Antioxidants and Fiber

by Sydney H. Crackower, M.D.,
Barry A. Bohn, M.D. and
Rodney Langlinais, Reg. Pharmacist

Intercontinental Marketing and Management
Lafayette, LA

One World Press
P.O. 2501
Prescott, AZ 86302

ISBN: 0-9644958-2-1

Library of Congress Number: 99-26939

Disclaimer: No information is this book is meant to replace professional medical consultation or treatment. In any matters related to your health please contact a qualified, licensed health practitioner.

Contents

One World Press
P.O. 2501
Prescott, AZ 86302

ISBN: 0-9644958-2-1

Library of Congress Number: 99-26939

Quantity Discounts Available

Preface

This book was written to help you realize the importance of good nutrition, i.e., the *wonderful* things that happen to your body if you are on a good nutritional diet and the bad things that happen if you aren't.

The two most important factors in nutrition are selectivity and consistency. Both the American Cancer Society and the American Heart Association have stated that if you eat five servings of fresh fruits and vegetables every day you lower the possibility of both heart attack and cancer by 55%. Consistently, by some means, everybody needs to get these fresh fruits and vegetables every day.

Selectivity is equally important. We need to choose the fruits and vegetables which optimally suit our nutritional needs...fruits and vegetables which contain the antioxidants, fiber and enzymes which are all essential to a healthy body.

If you improve your diet after reading this book, the effort to put it together will have been well worth it.

Sydney H. Crackower, M.D.
Barry Bohn, M.D.
Rodney Langlinais, Reg. Pharmacist

Introduction

The leading killer diseases of the latter part of this century are, without a doubt, vascular diseases (including heart attack and stroke) and cancer. Factors influencing vascular disease include diet, smoking, reduced physical activity, hypertension and diabetes. Factors influencing the risk of cancer include air and water pollution, diet, smoking, exposure to other airborne carcinogens and generic predisposition.

In recent years, research has pointed to the importance of a group of vitamins, minerals and nutrients called *antioxidants* which play significant roles in the prevention of these diseases.

When we cook our food we denature its enzyme content and also reduce the vitamin and mineral availability. Ideally, we should be consuming a diet that is raw in nature, instead of the refined, processed and cooked diet that we have all come to know and love.

Foods consumed in a raw state have the live, active enzymes intact. These enzymes assist our bodies in the breakdown of the foods we eat and therefore reduce the burden on our digestive organs. Again, when foods are cooked, refined and processed, the enzyme activity of these foods is greatly reduced, and in some cases nonexistent. This places a great burden on the digestive organs to produce adequate amounts of enzymes to break down proteins, carbohydrates and fats for all metabolic functions. This is particularly true for those who eat a "modern day" diet abundant in fat. Such a diet requires the pancreas to produce large amounts of lipase to break down fatty food substances.

Recent nutritional research has revealed the tremendous value of increasing fiber in the diet. This, of itself, will undoubtedly have a profound effect in the reduction of cancer of the colon and in the reduction of vascular disease. Again, heeding the timely advice of established health-promoting organizations, the consumption of five servings of fresh, raw fruit and vegetables on a daily basis will provide the fiber required to promote a reduction in the leading causes of death in modern civilization.

While the media has done an excellent job in providing the latest information concerning fat in the diet, the need for antioxidants and the importance of increased fiber, there still remain a number of nutrients and food "actives" found in fresh fruits and vegetables that will soon come to be known as potent disease fighters. Nutritional research into these nutrients will provide new weapons against AIDS, cancer, heart disease, arthritis, periodontal diseases and a variety of other ailments. Many new medical cures will be discovered in diets closer to nature—in fresh, uncooked fruits and vegetables.

1

ENZYMES

Enzymes are needed for every chemical action and reaction in the body. They act as energizing forces or catalysts. A chemical reaction which would otherwise take weeks or months is shortened to mere seconds by the work of an enzyme. (The rate at which an enzyme reacts is directly proportional to the concentration and availability of the enzyme.) Our organs, tissues and cells are run by metabolic enzymes. Minerals, vitamins and hormones need enzymes in order to do their work properly.

Enzymes are involved in every process of the body. Life could not exist without them. Enzymes digest all of our food, making it small enough to pass into the bloodstream through the minute pores of the intestines. Enzymes in the blood take prepared, digested food and build it into muscles, nerves, blood and glands. Enzymes are responsible for eliminating toxins from our lungs. The process whereby a sperm fertilizes an egg requires enzyme activity. Enzymes in our immune system attack foreign substances and toxins to rid the body of harmful invaders.

There are four categories of food enzymes, each with a specific function:

- Lipase breaks down fat,
- Protease breaks down protein,
- Cellulase breaks down cellulose,
- and Amylase breaks down starch.

Remembering the precise name of each enzyme is not important. What is important is that you understand how to get enzymes into your body, what their sources are, and that without them life would not exist. The more we become enzyme deficient, the faster we age. The more we store up our enzyme reserve, the healthier we will be.

There are two ways to preserve and replenish the enzyme level: 1. by eating raw food, and 2. by taking enzyme supplements. Let's talk about raw food first.

Live Food or Dead Food

The difference between live (raw) food and dead food is enzymatic activity. If you had two seeds and boiled one, which one would grow when placed in soil? There is no question that the unboiled seed would sprout because it has its enzymes intact.

We feed our bodies "dead" food when we cook it too long. This cooked food may taste delicious, but it lacks the great enzymatic energy which nature placed in it for our bodily functions.

Most enzymes function at an optimum temperature of 45 degrees C (only a few degrees above body temperature). Below 10 degrees C and above 60 degrees C, enzymes are inactive. Since enzymes cannot withstand the hot temperatures used in cooking, they are completely destroyed in all foods that are canned, pasteurized, baked, roasted, stewed, or fried.

A cooked food diet not only kills the enzymes in food but causes the endocrine glands to become overworked, thereby encouraging the development of diseases such as hypoglycemia and obesity. Cooked food raises the white blood cell count, can cause weight gain and also robs the body of enzymes which otherwise would have been used to maintain metabolism.

When we eat a diet of overcooked food we may be getting more than enough calories, but these calories may be "empty," i.e., lack the proper balance of nutrients and enzymes. In an effort to gain these necessary nutrients, the endocrine glands (which regulate appetite) may therefore overstimulate the digestive organs, demanding more food...much more than is needed to maintain strength and vitality. This results in over secretion of hormones, overeating, obesity and finally exhaustion of the hormone-producing glands...not to mention the depletion of enzyme reserves due to the increased metabolic activity. In a nutshell, when we steam, broil, fry, pasteurize, bake or microwave our food in any way we denature, or make ineffective, the natural enzymes contained in the food.

In older individuals, the enzyme content of the body has been depleted due to a lifetime of eating cooked foods which drain natural enzyme reserves. Moreover, lacking enzymes, the food is rarely digested properly and will ferment in the digestive tract producing toxins that are then absorbed into the blood and deposited in the joints and other soft-tissue areas.

Supplementation

Not everyone can or will eat a raw food diet, however. That is where enzyme supplementation, or a combination of supplementation and raw food, comes in. If one is sick or trying to recover either from an acute or chronic disease, taking enzymes supplements would be beneficial. A chronic disease is a disease that has lingered in the body for many weeks, months, or sometimes years. Such a disease becomes a constant drag on the body, depleting it of enzymes, vitamins, minerals and trace minerals. Thus, with chronic disease, there is usually a low body-reserve of enzymes. During all acute and chronic illnesses, enzymes are being used up more rapidly than is normal. People with hypoglycemia, endocrine gland deficiencies, obesity, anorexia nervosa and stress-related problems, could all benefit from enzyme supplementation.

Aging too correlates perfectly with the enzyme reserve in the body. A greater amount of enzymes are found in the young person's tissues than in an elderly person's tissues. Taking this into consideration, doing all you can to maintain and increase enzyme levels (both in the use of raw food and with supplementation) would be an advantage to tissue and organ longevity.

Enzymes and Aging

The truth is that age is not so much a matter of how many years one has been alive, but rather a matter of the integrity of the tissues of the body. (A sixty-year-old man or woman *can* have a body of someone in his or her forties.) Body tissues depend upon the amount of enzymes present to carry on the metabolism of every cell.

Our metabolism is maintained by enzyme activity. When our enzyme level is lowered, our metabolism is lowered and so is our energy level. As we have mentioned before, increasing age shows a slow decrease in the enzyme reserve. When the enzyme level becomes so low that metabolism itself is threatened, death results.

Any time the metabolism is falsely stimulated by coffee, a high protein diet or other stimulants, the metabolism increases and enzymes are quickly used up. This stimulation is accompanied by a false energy output, during which the individual feels a temporary sense of well-being. However, the end result will be lower energy (due to a more rapid burnout of enzymes). Over the long-term, this kind of consistent stimulation of metabolism results in premature old age.

Enzymes and Disease

Our immune system, bloodstream, liver, kidneys, spleen, pancreas, as well as our ability to see, think and breathe depend upon enzymes. Realizing that the lack of enzymes can be a predisposing factor in disease substantiates their importance. Enzymes break down toxic substances so that the body can eliminate them without damaging the eliminative organs. White blood cells provide transportation for enzymes throughout the body. The white blood cells help to destroy antigens and other toxins by engulfing them and then digesting or partially destroying their substance, making it easier for the body to eliminate them. White blood cells do this by secreting enzymes that break down the antigens. Yeast and most antigens can be eliminated by administering supplemental enzymes.

Good News For Athletes

An athlete's main concerns should be the types of food eaten in order to maintain a healthy body, and the replacement of nutrients which are lost during exercise or competition. Unfortunately, eating the proper quantities of foods and nutrients is only one half the issue. The other half is whether or not the athlete's system absorbs and properly utilizes the food ingested, since so many of our foods lack the proper enzymes. Nutrients may be present in the foods we eat, but the work-force of the body is in the enzymes. This is why most vitamins are called co-enzymes. This means that they must combine with enzymes before the body can use them.

Over-nutrition and under-absorption result in a low energy system. People often believe that they don't recover from exercise readily enough because they overdid it or didn't do enough. Actually, the problem may be that the body's "engine" is congested with unusable fuel, i.e., food that lacks enzymes.

Athletes need enzymes. Although the athlete may be taking vitamins, minerals and concentrated foods, it is enzymes that make all of these elements work. The utilization of vitamins depends upon enzymes, and enzymes often depend on vitamins. Under clinical observation it has been shown that, when taking vitamins which have been combined (in capsules) with enzymes, smaller amounts of vitamins and minerals are needed. Moreover, any time the body temperature is raised, as during exercise, enzymes are used up more rapidly than normal; carbohydrates are burned faster; and more nutrients are needed for fuel supplies. Since the athlete usually eats mostly cooked food, the situation is like burning the candle at both ends—enzymes are being used up rapidly and little is brought in to replenish the supply. Therefore, athletes can benefit by taking enzyme supplements.

Athletes who want to be able to work out more often and with greater intensity and less recovery time should depend upon enzymes. About half the amount of one's body energy is spent digesting food. If exogenous enzymes (taken through raw food or through supplementation) are added to the diet daily, more nutrients will be available and less food will be needed, resulting in less digestive stress and less waste elimination. This is precisely the type of energy conservation for health and stamina that athletes, and all of us, want and need!

2

FREE RADICALS, AGING AND CANCER

Generated by enzymatic and chemical reactions, *free radicals* form constantly in our body tissues and fluids as a normal consequence of metabolism. (Examples of free radicals are peroxides, epoxides and superoxides.) Free radicals are small molecules with an extra electron. This extra, unpaired electron causes the free radical molecule to move wildly and erratically throughout our tissues, looking for another electron to "steal" for its partner. In pairing, the electron strives to become more stable. The process of looking for an additional electron causes damage to any structure that the free radical bombards and to which it becomes attached. Free radical damage has been implicated in cancer, heart disease, aging, periodontal disease, cataracts, and Parkinson's disease. In fact, any inflammatory process probably has the free radical as an initiating force.

Free radicals are derived from numerous sources including air pollution, ultraviolet light, tobacco smoke and some medications. We are literally surrounded by free radicals, and it would appear that we have no protection from these potentially harmful molecules.

One substance that free radicals bombard, in an effort to attain an additional electron and thus become stable, is the DNA in the nuclei of our cells. When DNA molecules containing the genetic information of our cells are attacked by free radicals, their molecular structure is altered. What then happens to the altered DNA molecular is that it in turn becomes a free radical. The altered molecule then seeks, attacks and damages neighboring molecules. When the DNA of cells is changed, alterations occur and the genetic information of the cells is affected. The cells can then undergo changes leading to the formation of malignant cells which then grow at a different rate than neighboring cells not affected by free radicals. The rapid proliferation of these malignant cells then forms tumors within the tissues of our bodies.

What About Aging?

Again, free radicals attach themselves to whatever they can find. They may attack cell membranes, fat molecules or tissue linings. The chemical reaction that generates free radicals involves the metabolism of oxygen and other chemicals. What follows from the attack on membranes and other molecules by free radicals is tissue damage which produces aging. For example, the reason that exposure to ultraviolet radiation ages our skin is due to the formation of free radicals. So many people will compliment a woman on her beautiful complexion and the first thing they ask is what line of cosmetics she may use. Instead, what they should ask is how she is protecting against free radical damage. The answer may lie in her diet.

Nature had given us a protection against these harmful free radicals which appear to be everywhere and which threaten our state of health. That protection is found in a group of compounds called *antioxidants*. These compounds protect our cells by acting as scavengers for free radicals; binding to them, and carrying them out of the body. Antioxidants can appear in the form of enzymes, vitamins or minerals.

How do antioxidants work? They stop the free radical chain reaction by "giving up" their own electrons to pair with free radicals, thus effectively ending the harmful, erratic behavior that free radicals produce in damaging the cells, membranes, DNA and other molecules of our bodies.

The best-known of the antioxidants are vitamin A, beta carotene, vitamin C, vitamin E and selenium.

3

BETA-CAROTENE, PROMOTER OF HEALTHY BODIES

Beta-carotene is a provitamin (a substance that the body can transform into a vitamin) found in a wide variety of yellow- and orange-colored fruits and vegetables. (Technically, beta-carotene is actually a double molecule of vitamin A which can be converted to vitamin A in the intestines before absorption. Beta-carotene is also converted to vitamin A in the liver.)

Vitamin A defends cell membranes and tissue linings against the attack of free radicals by neutralizing the free radicals. Through their antioxidant effects, vitamin A and beta-carotene protect the body from the damaging effects of smoke and other pollutants, and may also play a role in preventing problems like ulcers, atherosclerosis (hardening of the arteries) and its complications, including high blood pressure and stroke. Beta-carotene helps to prevent arterial plaque which could be the cause of a stroke. Vitamin A is involved in forming new bone during growth and promoting healthy teeth.

By stimulation of the basal (lowest) layers of the skin's cells, vitamin A and beta-carotene help cells to form normally and give them their structural integrity. Vitamin A and beta-carotene do this not only for skin cells, but also for the mucus membrane linings of the nose, eyes, intestinal tract, respiratory lining and the bladder. In helping to protect these areas and by aiding in cell maturation in these areas, vitamin A and beta-carotene protect these areas from the development of cancer. Beta-carotene improves immune response by stimulating T-cell activity. (T-cells circulate in the blood and lymph and regulate the immune system's response to infected or malignant cells.) A number of studies have shown reduced lung and colon cancer rates in people with higher intakes of beta-carotene.

Vitamin A and beta-carotene help to protect tissues during infections and promote more rapid recovery, mainly through support of the health of the skin and mucus lining barriers. They stimulate the production of mucus and improve antibody response and white cell functions. They help prevent the irritating effects of smoke and pollution.

Beta-carotene is found in kale, parsley, lettuce, broccoli, spinach, carrots, apricots, peaches, papaya, mango, and cantaloupe.

Vitamin A, besides its antioxidant effect, is essential for eyesight because of its formation of rhodopsin, or visual purple, which allows us to have night vision. Night blindness is found in individuals lacking sufficient vitamin A as the visual purple must be regenerated. Vitamin A is used in the compound *Retin A*, now used in medicine to treat acne and wrinkles. Vitamin A is also used for wound healing following surgery.

In summary, provitamin A, or beta-carotene and vitamin A, maintain the integrity of tissues in the body and aid in cancer prevention by acting as antioxidants which behave as scavengers of free radicals. The best sources of these antioxidants appear to be fruits and vegetables, mainly of the yellow and orange varieties. Dark green vegetables also provide a rich source of vitamin A.

4

VITAMIN C—FOR SUPPORT AND SHAPE

Vitamin C must be obtained from the diet; this puts Vitamin C in the category of being an essential nutrient. Vitamin C is found only in fresh fruits and vegetables; in highest quantity in fresh, uncooked foods. A deficiency of vitamin C can cause the disease known as *scurvy*—a condition which causes bleeding disorders, gum inflammation, weakness and tooth decay. First written about around 1500 B.C., scurvy was described by Aristotle, in 450 B.C.. Over the centuries it was found that the juice of lemons could cure and prevent this disease. The chemical name for vitamin C is *ascorbic acid*.

When absorbed from the intestine, vitamin C is used up by the body in two hours. Thus, to maintain the body's necessary level of vitamin C, fruits and vegetables should ideally be eaten several times a day. Vitamin C is used up even more rapidly under stressful conditions, especially with alcohol and tobacco use. The blood levels of this vitamin are lower in smokers than in nonsmokers. Other conditions that reduce absorption of vitamin C or increase utilization include:

- fever,
- viral illnesses,
- the use of antibiotics, aspirin and cortisone

- and exposure to environmental toxins such as petroleum products and DDT.

Vitamin C tends to be stored in the adrenal glands, ovaries, testes, and the eyes. To maintain body stores, we need a minimum of 200 mg. a day in our diet. Much more is needed if we are under stress, consume alcohol, smoke, or have diabetes.

The best known sources of vitamin C are the citrus fruits—oranges, lemons, limes, tangerines and grapefruits. The fruits with the highest natural concentrations include papaya, acerola cherries, cantaloupes and strawberries. The best known vegetable sources of vitamin C are red and green peppers, broccoli, brussels sprouts, tomatoes, asparagus, parsley, cabbage and dark green, leafy vegetables.

Vitamin C is important in the formation and support of collagen (the building block of connective tissue). Collagen is found in skin, ligaments, cartilage, the vertebrae of the spine, as well as in bones and teeth. Vitamin C is required, therefore, to give shape and support to our bodies, to maintain healthy blood vessels and to help in wound healing.

Vitamin C is also needed in the formation of brain chemicals. Vitamin C stimulates adrenal function and the release of adrenaline in times of stress. It aids in thyroid hormone production and assists in helping the body to eliminate cholesterol. As an antioxidant vitamin, ascorbic acid or vitamin C helps prevent oxidation of water-soluble molecules that would otherwise form free radicals and cause cellular damage and disease. Vitamin C detoxifies substances produced from the drugs cortisone, insulin and aspirin.

Recent research reveals that this vitamin plays a role in immune function and thus helps in the prevention of infections. Ascorbic acid appears to activate the white blood cells, the neutrophils, which are the front line defense against infectious diseases. Vitamin C also increases the production of lymphocytes, the cells important in antibody formation. The anti-viral substance *interferon* is positively influenced in production by the presence of sufficient amounts of vitamin C. Because of its healing properties, vitamin C has been used by physicians in treating burns, fractures, bedsores and other skin ulcers, and to speed wound healing after surgery. Through its antioxidant effect, vitamin C reduces the damage caused by pollution. Some recent reports indicate that vitamin C may be helpful in the prevention of glaucoma and cataract formations mainly through its antioxidant properties.

Because it reduces platelet aggregation, a factor important in the prevention of plaque in hardening of the arteries, vitamin C appears to play an important role in preventing coronary artery disease and stroke. Due to its antioxidant effect, vitamin C will no doubt soon play an important role in reducing the risk of cancer.

The many functions of this important vitamin underline the importance of eating the five servings of raw fruits and vegetables suggested by the American Cancer Society and the National Cancer Institute. There is little doubt that fruits and vegetables, by virtue of their antioxidant content, provide significant risk reduction in the development of cancer.

5

VITAMIN E—THE MOST VERSATILE ANTIOXIDANT

Vitamin E is a fat-soluble vitamin comprised of a family of compounds known as *tocopherols*. Although there is no known deficiency disease involving vitamin E, it is an essential vitamin.

Our diets today are generally low in vitamin E. It is most abundant in many "frying" oils which are so high in cholesterol that they have become less popular for many people today because of concern about heart disease. Moreover, in the process of refining and purifying vegetable oils much of the vitamin E is lost.

Vitamin E is absorbed from the small intestine with fat and bile salts. First it enters the lymphatic system, then moves on to the bloodstream, finally to be stored in the liver, the fatty tissues and the heart. Vitamin E is also found in the uterus, ovaries, adrenal glands, testes and muscles. Estrogen supplements and unsaturated oil cause vitamin E to become depleted.

The best sources of vitamin E are brussels sprouts, leafy green vegetables, spinach, soybeans, whole wheat and whole-grain cereals. It is also found in kale, spinach and tomatoes.

The main function of vitamin E is its antioxidant activity. When saturated fats, rancid oils, hydrogenated oils and polyunsaturated fats become oxidized (the addition of oxygen causes electrons to be "knocked loose"), free radicals are released which lead to cellular and tissue damage. This in turn leads to an inflammatory process in the linings of blood vessels. From this process we get such diseases as hardening of the arteries (atherosclerosis), high blood pressure, arthritis, and some forms of cancer. Vitamin E is able to protect our tissues from the oxidation effects of free radicals.

The frying of foods in oil creates many oxidized by-products of fat. This makes the consumption of fried foods hazardous in our daily diets.

Vitamin E serves to stabilize cell membranes. It protects the lungs from oxidative damage due to harmful substances in our environment. Vitamin E also preserves the biological action of vitamin A, another important fat-soluble vitamin. Generally speaking, vitamin E stabilizes the lipids (fats) in the blood so that the heart, blood vessels and other structures are protected from injury induced by free radicals.

For many years now, the anti-clotting effects of vitamin E have been well known. The respiration of heart and muscle cells is improved by the utilization of less oxygen by these tissues, which happens in the presence of vitamin E. This, in turn, improves endurance and stamina, and reduces heart disease. More recently, vitamin E has been shown to reduce the sticking together of the platelets of the blood and their adhesiveness to the walls of blood vessels. All of this would tend to make vitamin E prevent the blockages we see in coronary artery disease and stroke, as well as the blockages in the vessels of the legs and feet.

An as antioxidant, vitamin E also enhances circulation and oxygenation. Current research tends to indicate that the skin changes associated with aging may be brought about by free radical damage. Vitamin E taken in amounts exceeding 100 I.U. per day, and between 100 and 400 I.U., has been shown to reduce coronary artery disease by interfering with the cholesterol molecules in their formation of the plaque which builds up in coronary arteries, as well as cerebral and peripheral blood vessels. Thus, vitamin E apparently plays a vital role in disease prevention.

Recent research has shown that laboratory rats receiving adequate supplements of vitamin E could tolerate higher ozone levels than rats which did not receive vitamin E supplementation.

Much research into the beneficial effects of vitamin E is still ongoing. To date, this antioxidant has been shown to be of the utmost importance in preventing disease by reducing cellular and tissue damage. Because our diets do not provide adequate amounts of vitamin E, it behooves us to obtain this important antioxidant by eating the vegetable products previously mentioned in this chapter.

6

SELENIUM—
A TRACE MINERAL

Selenium, a trace element, is absolutely necessary for metabolism. It functions as part of an enzyme called *glutathione peroxidase,* and because of this association, selenium plays an important role in preventing cancer and cardiovascular disease.

Whenever there are low soil levels of selenium, there are increased cancer rates. Whenever the soil is rich in selenium, there are below-average cancer rates; particularly cancer of the breast, lungs and colon. In Keshan, China, many children suffer from a disease which causes an enlarged heart and congestive heart failure. However, this disease responds positively to selenium treatment. The soil of this part of China is deficient in the mineral selenium. In the United States, South Dakota has the highest selenium concentration; Ohio has the lowest. The result is that Ohio has more than twice the number of cancer cases than South Dakota.

Selenium and vitamin E work together as antioxidants. Together they do a better job of stimulating the immune system than they do independently. Most of the selenium found in our bodies is found in the liver, kidneys and pancreas; and in men, in the testes and seminal vesicles.

The amount of selenium found in meats, fruits and vegetables varies from region to region depending on the selenium content of the soil. Rich sources of selenium include barley, oats, whole wheat, brown rice, broccoli, garlic, onions, mushrooms, tomatoes, radishes, shellfish, Brazil nuts, liver, fish and lamb.

Selenium is known to help prevent cardiovascular disease and to decrease the risk of complications such as strokes and heart attacks, most likely by reducing the "sticking together" or aggregation of blood platelets. In animal studies the addition of one to four parts per million of selenium, added to food or water, reduces cancer rates. High breast cancer rates are found in areas with a low concentration of selenium in the soil. These epidemiological studies cannot be overlooked or ignored. Selenium appears to be a most important mineral in the prevention of cancer and cardiovascular disease.

7

FIBER AND YOUR DIGESTIVE SYSTEM

Overview

For many years we have known that fiber is beneficial to human beings and their digestive systems. Fiber is essential, but unfortunately most Americans eat only one-third of the fiber they need on a daily basis. Most of us need to increase our dietary fiber intake to 25–30 grams per day.

The National Cancer Institute has recommended reduction of fat consumption and increased fiber consumption in the American diet. This is feasible but difficult to accomplish. The relationship between food groups and nutrient intake (specifically fiber and vegetables and fruits) is apparently related to household income, ethnicity and residence throughout the country. Educating the public to increase consumption of both fiber and fruits and vegetables will take a concerted national effort.

Epidemiologic studies have shown that colon rectal cancer is a major public health issue in North America and Western Europe, and seems to be increasing in many other areas of the world as well. Increased dietary levels of fiber, vitamin C and beta-carotene could possibly decrease this risk. Studies of colon rectal cancer show a decreased risk as the fiber intake increases. Estimates are that the 50,000 cases of this particular cancer reported annually could be reduced about 30% by increasing the average fiber intake in food sources to 25 grams per day. Dietary factors play a key role in the prevention of large bowel cancer. Here too a diet of 25% fat and 25 grams of fiber is recommended.

Attempts to increase dietary fiber intake, however beneficial, need to address the expectations, attitudes and beliefs of certain social structures and social status. Food choices, diet, and social status are highly related and many of these will require early childhood education to alter lifelong behavior. Comprehensive school health education will be needed to modify the nutritional habits of children in this country. So, teach your children well.

Fiber and Cholesterol

Several types of soluble and insoluble fiber influence the level of cholesterol and triglycerides in the blood. Soluble fiber such as oat bran is known to decrease total cholesterol levels. Women over fifty with high cholesterol levels seem to respond nicely to oat bran dietary supplementation.

It is well known that supplementation of the diet with a soluble fiber reduces cholesterol beyond the reduction observed with just a low fat diet. Oat bran appears to have some beneficial effect on cholesterol by increasing the HDL cholesterol, which is the "good" type of cholesterol. Oat bran also assists in reducing the ratio of LDL-C to HDL-C. This ratio reduction is important to humans.

Depending on the genetic makeup of certain individuals, oat bran fiber supplementation seems to have an advantage over wheat bran fiber in significantly lowering the LDL or the "bad" cholesterol. Some patients who have been placed on a high fiber diet showed a significant weight loss and drop in blood cholesterol level also. Exactly how oat bran produces lowering of cholesterol is not quite known. It is a soluble fiber and is broken down in the colon into chemicals called short chain fatty acids (SCFAs). These SCFAs may have something to do with cholesterol synthesis.

Barley, another soluble dietary fiber, seems to have a definite hypocholesterolemic effect in certain animal studies, especially in young chickens. Also, barley contains beta-glucan as a source of soluble dietary fiber and appears to be more effective than wheat fiber at lowering blood cholesterol in men with high blood cholesterol levels.

Another type of fiber, called glucomannan, has been shown to have a beneficial effect in obese and abnormally fat-laden children when combined with a low fat diet. Excess weight and triglycerides were significantly decreased in these children when glucomannan studies were done. Other studies indicate that glucomannan seems to improve the lipid status and carbohydrate tolerance.

One form of pectin, a water soluble dietary fiber, may be a useful adjunct to the diet in the management of higher plasma cholesterol.

Some fruits, such as guava, can possibly cause a substantial reduction of blood pressure and blood fats, without decreasing the "good" cholesterol (the HDL cholesterol) due to their soluble fiber content.

Among desert nomads in certain countries, fiber from beets has been shown to provide an alternative effective therapy for control of elevated cholesterol levels.

Prune fiber seems to significantly lower low density lipoprotein LDL cholesterol.

Fiber and Coronary Disease

High fiber diets have been associated with a reduced incidence of coronary heart disease. Studies are underway on antioxidant vitamins and their association with a reduced incidence of coronary heart disease, as well. Diet is a key factor which modifies both the blood and antioxidant levels. It has been recommended by some that a diet high in fiber and high in antioxidant vitamins (beta-carotene seems to be protective and puts people in a lower risk category) may reduce the risk of coronary heart disease, particularly in men. Fiber seems to be equally protective in both sexes. There is a favorable long-term effect of a low fat, high fiber diet on the way that human blood coagulates and the way that clots are broken up. It appears that a low fat, high fiber diet produces an increase in a plasma fraction of the blood that has a beneficial activity related to the adhesion of fibrin clots. This has a favorable effect, reducing cardiovascular risks in humans.

Soluble oat fiber can significantly lower plasma total cholesterol and LDL cholesterol, and thus potentially lower the risk of coronary heart disease. Also, apple pectin mixed with other fiber in a soft drink seems to have beneficial effects on some patients at risk with coronary heart disease.

Dietary intake of fiber is related to hypertension. Those on a high fiber, low fat and low sodium diet have a much better chance of reducing or even stopping their medications for hypertension.

Fiber and Cancer
Colon cancer
In the Western world, the common high fat, low fiber food diet is related to the increased risk of cancer in the colon, pancreas, breast, prostate, ovary and endometrium. Increased dietary fiber reduces this risk. Certain chemicals produced during the cooking of meat (heterocyclic amines) may be carcinogens. When fiber is digested by bacteria in the colon, short chain fatty acids are produced. One of these (butyrate) has anti-cancer effects on human colon and rectal cancer cells. Short chain fatty acids also have a beneficial effect for the colon in regards to its immune function. This may explain the decreased incidence in colon rectal cancer in those with high fiber diets.

Another interesting association between the amount of dietary fiber and the removal of certain chemicals from the colon follows: In human feces, the high dietary intake of fiber may actually increase a chemical called *fecapentaene*. One component of this chemical may actually adhere to dietary fiber and be removed from the body. This removal appears to be related to some effects of that particular chemical which may relate to formation of colon cancer.

In 1971, Denis Burkitt announced his hypothesis that a fiber depleted diet was a cause of colon rectal cancer. He based his thesis on observations of the differences in the diets of people in Western countries contrasted to those within traditional African societies. Subsequent studies have verified some of his hypothesis showing that a high fiber diet has a definite protective effect, i.e., reduction of colon rectal cancer.

Rates of colon and rectal cancers in various countries are strongly related with per-capita consumption of red meat and animal fat, and inversely associated with fiber consumption. A high intake of fiber—including vegetables, fruits and grains—coupled with a low intake of saturated fat is associated with a decreased risk of polyps and tumors of the colon.

Fiber puts females in a lower risk category for colon cancer, while certain types of fat put them at higher risk. The risk of colon rectal cancer is decreased with the intake of grain fiber for both females and males. For males, some studies have shown that high intake of soluble grain fiber appeared to be associated with lower risk. For rectal cancers, increased intake of fruit and vegetable fiber is associated with decreased risk.

Bacteria in the colon secrete and produce certain types of enzymes in the bowel, and these enzymes seem to have some relationship to the production of colon cancer. In certain studies, consumption of oat bran as a dietary fiber had a beneficial effect in decreasing some of these particular enzymes. This may explain oat bran's beneficial effect in reducing the incidence of cancer of the colon. It is believed that some dietary fibers actually adhere to or assist in adsorbing some of the chemicals which are cancer causing agents. Studies in Argentina have shown that dietary fiber is highly protective in relation to the incidence of colon cancer. Both human and animal studies suggest a tumor-promoting role of bile acids in the development of colon tumors. Human studies seem to be somewhat conflicting. Pectin is another type of fiber found in many fruits and vegetables. Supplementation of the diet (especially in some animals) with 10% pectin has been found to suppress colon cancer to a significant extent.

Breast cancer
Apparently, fiber in the diet is associated with a reduction in the incidence of breast cancer and has some protective effects. Fiber may modify those risks of breast cancer which are associated with the American high fat, low fiber diet. These effects may be the result of certain chemicals called *phytoestrogens* (plant type estrogens) which decrease the incidence of breast cancer.

Women who had higher intakes of dietary fiber had a 30% reduction in risk of breast cancer as opposed to women who had the lowest intake of fiber.

Fiber and Other Diseases
Dietary fiber also seems beneficial in other diseases such as diabetes mellitus and Parkinsonism. It is believed by some that addition of fiber to the diet of diabetic patients may even prevent or delay vascular complications. Because diabetics must limit their intake of foods that are high in fats or sugars, the addition of foods with fiber is beneficial to this population. Moreover, a diet higher in fiber may also help with compliance, perhaps because it gives the patient a sense of satisfaction or fullness.

Interestingly, diets which are rich in soluble fiber seem to be of assistance in treating patients with Parkinson's disease who are currently taking one of its main medications, L-dopa.

Summary

Dietary fiber has many benefits. These generally relate to cholesterol, vascular disease, colon rectal cancer, breast cancer, diabetes and other diseases. Everyone is encouraged to increase intake of fiber to 25–30 grams per day especially by increasing the daily intake of vegetables, fruits and grain.

8

PHYTOCHEMICALS

When you think about whether you're eating a healthy diet you probably worry about getting sufficient vitamins and minerals. But, do you ever wonder if you are getting the proper phytochemicals? Phytochemicals are compounds that give plant foods their color, odor and flavor; they also contribute to a plant's self-defense system. Each phytochemical has a different name, such as *capsaicin* in hot peppers. Phytochemicals are the hottest news in nutrition— they boast a long list of health benefits! Some phytochemicals may help prevent cancer and other serious ailments.

Because phytochemicals are present in all fruits and vegetables and many other common plant foods, it is easy to work them into your diet. You can get these healthful substances from whole grains, beans, peas and many herbs and spices, too.

Scientists are discovering that many phytochemicals seem to be preventing various types of cancer in animals. They appear to work almost like magic by interfering with the development of cancer at the cellular level. Some phytochemicals prevent cancer-causing chemicals from forming; others protect cells from damage.

Cancer is not the only target of these nutritional weapons. Some phytochemicals may forestall diabetes, while others block infectious diseases by boosting the immune system. Still others appear to reduce the risk of heart disease.

Seven important and well-researched food sources that contain phytochemicals significant to health are:

1. Garlic: which contains *allium*. This phytochemical may lower cholesterol and may block the formation of cancer causing chemicals.

2. Hot peppers: which contain *capsaicin*, which may short-circuit the development of various types of cancer; capsaicin helps to prevent toxic substances from attaching to the DNA within the body cells.

3. Carrots: which contain *carotenoids* (also found in sweet potatoes, cantaloupe, parsley, spinach and cauliflower). Carotenoids may stave off lung cancer by shielding the cells from toxins.

4. Tomatoes: which contain *coumarins* also found in citrus fruits. These phytochemicals may stop the body from forming substances that can give rise to cancer and may prevent blood clots.

5. Kale: which contains *indoles* (also found in brussels sprouts, cabbage and broccoli). Indoles may protect against a variety of cancers by making dangerous toxins easier to excrete.

6. Oranges: which contain *limonoid* (also found in other citrus fruits). They may stimulate the production of natural substances that break down many cancer-causing chemicals.

7. Raspberries: which contain *phenols* (also found in grapes, strawberries and blueberries). Phenols may reduce the risk of cancer by trapping toxic chemicals and flushing them out of the body.

9

B COMPLEX—THE GREAT ENERGIZING FORCE OF THE BODY

The group of vitamins referred to as B complex are a group of water-soluble vitamins which are not stored well in the body. For this reason, they are required on a daily basis to support many body functions. They are called *B complex* because they are found together in foods and have similar coenzyme (enzyme-helping) functions.

The microorganisms in our bodies can actually *make* B vitamins in our intestines. The B vitamins are absorbed into the bloodstream from the small intestine. There are many B-vitamin deficiency diseases, but little or no toxic effects of B vitamins.

The B group of vitamins are found in Brewer's yeast, many vegetables, whole wheat, bran, milk, lean pork, organic meats, fish and eggs. Other sources include cabbage, cantaloupe, soy beans, and walnuts.

Vitamin B 1, also known as *thiamine*, has a key role in the cellular production of energy. It helps convert carbohydrates to fat, a process needed to produce energy. Thiamine is important in the nervous system due to its role in making the neurotransmitter, acetylcholine. When B 1 is deficient, there appears to be more inflammatory activity in nervous tissue. Thiamine plays a role in the learning capacity and growth of children.

Vitamin B 2, known as *riboflavin*, is easily absorbed from the small intestine into the bloodstream and then into the tissues. Riboflavin functions as a building block for two coenzymes important in energy production. It is also important in cell respiration, helping cells use oxygen in an efficient manner. Riboflavin is important to vision and healthy hair, nails and skin.

Vitamin B 3, called *niacin*, is involved in more than fifty different metabolic reactions. Many of these reactions involve extracting energy from carbohydrates and glucose. It is also involved in the production of red blood cells and the metabolism of some drugs and toxic substances. The coenzymes of niacin break down proteins, fats and carbohydrates. Niacin also promotes circulation and reduces cholesterol in the blood. This vitamin is also used in the synthesis of sex hormones, such as estrogen, testosterone and progesterone.

Vitamin B 5, *pantothenic acid*, functions as part of a molecule called Coenzyme A (CoA). As CoA is involved in the function of the adrenal cortex, it is known as the "anti-stress" vitamin. The adrenal glands secrete cortisone and other hormones when the body is stressed. Pantothenic acid improves the health and appearance of nerves and skin structures. By this activity, vitamin B 5 may slow the process of aging and the formation of wrinkles.

The overall metabolic importance of Vitamin B 5 is in the metabolism of carbohydrates and fats for the release of energy. As a coenzyme, B 5 is involved in the synthesis of the chemical nerve messenger, acetylcholine, the agent that permits the innervation (growth of nerves) within muscles.

Vitamin B 6, or *pyridoxine*, is important in protein metabolism. When protein is broken down into amino acids,

B 6 aids in the transport of the amino acids into the bloodstream and from the blood into the cells.

During pregnancy, vitamin B 6 functions to maintain a hormonal balance in the mother, and plays an important role in the development of the nervous system of the developing baby.

B 12, or *cobalamin*, was isolated in 1926 when it was discovered that its deficiency caused pernicious anemia. (This disease causes a degeneration of the nervous system.) For absorption, vitamin B 12 requires the production of an "intrinsic factor" found in the mucus secretion of the stomach. Elderly people often do not produce this factor adequately, and, therefore, often have a B 12 deficiency. The important function of this vitamin is in maintaining the health of the nervous system and in the metabolism of nerve tissue. The vitamin stimulates growth in children and is needed in the manufacture of red blood cells by the body.

The reason many patients find that an injection of B 12 gives them a burst of energy is because the vitamin increases the utilization of carbohydrates, proteins, and fats by the body.

The entire group of B vitamins are essentially the "batteries" of the body, providing an important source of energy for countless metabolic reactions.

10

CATARACTS AND FRESH FRUITS AND VEGETABLES

The health literature is replete with references to the consumption of fruits, vegetables and various antioxidant vitamins in relationship to cataract formation. Recent studies suggest that a diet low in vitamin E is a risk factor in the formation of cataracts. Those patients with higher blood levels of vitamin E seem to have a reduced risk for various types of cataract development.

Some physicians have recommended that ophthalmologists join other health care professionals, wellness professionals and prevention professionals in helping their patients change their lifestyles to choose a diet which is heavy in antioxidants, specifically vitamins C and E. In addition, cutting down on smoking, which certainly raises the risk of cataracts in many different studies, is highly recommended. Smokers are more than twice as likely to develop cataracts as non-smokers; and the risk of development of cataracts increases with the number of cigarettes smoked.

People who work outdoors (especially in equatorial zones of the world), work on the water, or work constantly at high altitudes should try to protect their eyes from excessive sunlight. Sunlight exposure is now well recognized as a factor in cataract development.

The consumption of large amounts of raw uncooked spinach has been associated with a lower relative risk for the development of cataracts. The risk of cataract development is much lower among women who use vitamin C in their diets for ten years or more.

Conclusions are that dietary carotenoids and long-term vitamin C usage may significantly decrease the risk of cataracts. Dietary intake of riboflavin, vitamins C, E, and beta carotene (which are antioxidants), protect against the development of the different types of cataracts. Occupational exposure to sunlight and smoking are definitely factors which increase the development of cataracts. Epidemiologists have found that cataract patients tend to have lower blood serum levels of vitamin C, E or carotenoids.

Randomized studies done in Hong Kong fishing communities in 1989 give support to the hypothesis that sunlight causes cataracts, again demonstrating the necessity of protecting your eyes with some sort of sunglasses, especially if you have an outdoor occupation.

The antioxidant vitamins, which are present in fruits and vegetables, are tremendously important. People who consume fewer than three and a half servings of raw uncooked fruits or vegetables per day have an increased risk of cataract development.

Cataract development research is also currently concentrating on oxygen free radicals in the bloodstream and in the ocular lens. The facts relating to their causing cataracts and the methods by which this happens are being studied intensively. Scavenging antioxidant vitamins found in many fruits and vegetables may be useful in preventing this particular problem. It is well known that vitamin E is one of the most effective chain-breaking antioxidants available. Vitamin E shows promise as a protective agent in preventing and minimizing oxygen free radicals which may be associated with cataracts, cancer, aging, circulatory conditions and arthritis, among other conditions.

Patients with chronic kidney failure and diminished levels of vitamin E in their blood seem to be at a relatively high risk for the development of cataracts. Recent discoveries indicate that vitamin E should be avoided in retinitis pigmentosa. Certain specific types of vitamin A in high doses are recommended in that particular disorder. In summary, five servings a day of raw uncooked fruits and vegetables, especially those containing vitamins A, C, and E, seem to be extremely beneficial in placing patients in a low risk category for developing several different types of cataracts. Much research is still being done at this time to find out more specifics.

11

AGING OF THE RETINA

The retina is the lining that covers the internal part of the eye; a layer that essentially covers the back two-thirds of the eye. The retina is responsible for transmitting images of light to the optic nerve and thus to the brain, where they are interpreted.

The retina is like the film in a camera. When it does not function properly the image of what we see is blurred, distorted or malformed. Embryologically, it is part of the nervous system and as such is very complex in its structure. The retina is sensitive to insults and yet resilient. It is subject to damage from many different diseases. One of these is called *Age Related Macular Degeneration* (abbreviated as ARMD hereafter).

The *macula* is the small central part of the retina which comprises only a small percent of the entire retinal surface. The macula is highly specialized and contains specialized cells called *cones* in high concentration. These cones enable us to have good visual acuity. If the macula is damaged, our ability to read, drive, sew, perform detailed work and watch TV is impaired.

One of the most common causes of legal blindness is ARMD. This is true for much of the modern world. Legal blindness means you are unable to read any of the large letters on an eye chart. Generally ARMD never causes complete blindness or absence of all vision. However, it is an extremely common condition especially in those over sixty years of age. Many of these patients must cease driving and many undergo extreme psychological difficulties in coping with the loss of independence that is associated with losing a driver's license. Although they may retain hope and benefit from various types of large-print books, magnifiers, telescopes, low vision devices and new costly computers, many remain restless, depressed, confused and frustrated by this condition.

ARMD is one of two types, dry or wet. The dry type is essentially an atrophic or nonvascular degeneration of the macula. This is the most common type and accounts for about 90% of cases. The wet type is associated with new, unwanted blood vessels (called subretinal neovascularization) which grow and proliferate in the macula and create havoc in its structure and function. This type, fortunately, only comprises 10% or so of all ARMD cases.

The cause of ARMD is complex. Heredity undoubtedly plays a part. Blue-eyed blondes seem to have a greater risk of developing this condition. It is more common in some races and some families. Its frequency increases with increasing age, especially over seventy-five years.

It is well know that smokers are at higher risk for developing ARMD and its associated loss of independence with aging. Just as cigarettes produce free radicals and oxidation products inducing changes in the human lens (cataracts), so do they contribute to the causation of ARMD.

Excessive exposure to blue light with a short wave length is also another factor which contributes to ARMD. Toxic free radical formation produced by exposure to blue light is a major factor in ARMD. Those who have a high exposure to sunlight throughout their lives and who do not use blue-blocker sun protection are at high risk for ARMD.

Another curious finding is that people with a weak handgrip strength seem to have a greater risk of ARMD. It is interesting that studies in vegetarians and Seventh Day

Adventists (also vegetarians) have shown they have a much stronger handgrip strength. Athletes who consume high quantities of fruits and vegetables have a greater handgrip strength. There are thus several factors which can be modified to reduce the risk of ARMD. (These would not include changing your hereditary status or race at this point.) Ceasing to smoke appears obvious. Wearing protective eye wear which blocks shortwave blue light is simple and recommended especially for those with a strong family history and those who work outdoors, on the water, in the mountains, etc.

Another good plan for reducing your risk of ARMD is to increase your consumption of raw uncooked fruits and vegetables to five servings a day. The rest of this book is devoted to reasons why you should be doing that anyway. Those reasons pertain to many aspects of your health far more important to your longevity than ARMD. However, since compliance is a problem which most researchers have noticed, much research is currently centered on the use of specific antioxidants, zinc, selenium, and supplements specifically related to ARMD. There still remains much controversy as to their effectiveness and how they work with this condition. Scientists are conducting many studies to analyze which component of the diet is most critical to decreasing your risk for ARMD. These studies may take many years and will undoubtedly be somewhat confusing for the average person to interpret. In the meantime, increase your consumption of raw fruits and vegetables to five times a day, or consume as much *fresh* fruit and vegetable juice as practical, or seek other alternatives if available.

12

CRANBERRY

Cranberry juice has long been recommended in certain types of kidney problems and urinary tract infection. Juice from the cranberry (a plant of the vaccinium genus Ericaceae) inhibits the adhesions of certain types of bacteria in the urinary system. The main effect of cranberry juice in the bladder and other areas of the body is in preventing infections.

During the mid-1800s, German physicians observed that the urinary excretion of hippuric acid (a bacteriostatic agent in high concentrations) increased after the ingestion of cranberries. It was believed that cranberries, prunes and plums contained benzoic acid or some other compound that the body metabolized and excreted as hippuric acid. This hypothesis has always been disputed because the amounts of benzoic acid present in these fruits (about 0.1% by weight) could not account for the excretion of the larger amounts of hippuric acid. It is likely that cranberry juice does not exert a directed antibacterial effect via a compound such as hippuric acid. Rather, that an alternate mechanism accounts for the anti-infective activity: Cranberry and blueberry juices contain a high molecular-weight-compound that inhibits the common urinary pathogen, Escherichia coli, from adhering to infection sites within the urinary tract, thereby limiting the ability of the bacteria to initiate and spread infections.

One promising use for cranberry juice is as a "urinary deodorant." The odor of fermenting urine from incontinent patients is a persistent, demoralizing problem in hospitals and long-term care facilities. Cranberry juice appears to lower urinary pH sufficiently to retard the degradation of urine by E. coli, limiting the generation of the pungent ammoniacal odor.

Using cranberry juice in combination with antibiotics has been suggested for the long-term suppressive therapy of urinary tract infections. Anecdotal reports have described the benefits of drinking six ounces of juice twice daily to relieve symptoms of chronic pyelonephritis (inflammation of the kidney and its pelvis, caused by bacterial infection), and to decrease the recurrence of urinary stones. The juice shows slight antiviral activity in vitro.

13

PAY ATTENTION TO CATECHINS

Catechins are interesting compounds; polyphenol catechins are predominately complex chemicals which are found in various types of food, and in Chinese green tea in particular. Chinese green tea is the most popular and commonly consumed beverage in many countries of the Eastern world.

Research regarding catechin derivatives shows that polyphenol catechins have many interesting and beneficial aspects for humans. Some of the components of this particular chemical inhibit the activity of the HIV-1 RT virus (immunodeficiency virus type 1, reverse transcriptase). This may have some important benefits in certain patients with this immunodeficiency virus, and additional studies are underway at this time.

Catechin derivatives also seem to inhibit Hepatitis B virus replication in certain chemical situations. Other aspects of catechin derivatives relate to the inhibition of the infective properties of the Herpes simplex virus.

Chromosomal damage caused by different types of cancer-causing agents is inhibited by certain types of catechin compounds, both in bacteria and in mammals. These catechins may be useful in the prevention of some types of cancer.

Some of the beneficial activities of catechins may be explained by their scavenging effect on free radicals which constantly roam the body. Some studies suggest that the catechins affect cancer during the stage in which the tumor is actually being promoted by certain cellular and tissue mechanisms. This antioxidant activity is directed toward such chemicals as hydrogen peroxide (H_2O_2) and the superoxide radical (O_2-). Catechins acting in this antioxidant way appear to interfere with tumor promotion and cell death. Also, catechins cut down on the intracellular communications of cancer-promoting chemicals.

Certain derivatives of catechins could provide effects against a wide spectrum of skin tumor promoters. Some types of skin tumors caused by certain chemical promoters are inhibited, blocked or interfered with by catechin consumption.

Green tea has been found to act positively by damaging certain harmful bacterial membranes. In some studies, polyphenol catechins were also found to inhibit and decrease the production and synthesis of DNA in certain rat liver tumor cells. Many anti-cancer effects of polyphenol catechins are being found in both human and animal research. Some researchers believe that polyphenol catechins are very useful as practical, cancer-prevention agents available in everyday life. These particular chemicals are non-toxic. Other studies suggest that polyphenol catechins cut down on gastric secretion and fight certain effects in the stomach which produce ulcers. This is caused primarily by their action of inhibiting certain gastric enzymes. Curiously, the polyphenol catechins are also reported to possess some protective activities against the cholera bacteria, perhaps because of their cellular membrane activities on the bacteria membrane.

Polyphenol catechins have a beneficial effect on reducing the blood coagulation process, increasing the breakup of fiber and clots, helping with the prevention of platelet clumping and adhesions, and decreasing cholesterol counts in human large blood vessels. It is felt by some that this is a type of prevention for hardening of the arteries.

Another benefit seems to be definite antimicrobial and catechin-microbicidal activities against mycoplasma (one of the major causes of pneumonia). A certain extract of catechins has shown a marked activity in killing the pneumonia bacteria. Catechins might be used, therefore, as a preventive measure against mycoplasma pneumonia infections.

In summary, the polyphenol catechins appear to be powerful antioxidant agents found in green tea extracts, and have been long used by many people in the Asian world. They are beneficial chemicals for antimicrobial activity against various types of bacteria, act as scavengers in the process of removing free radicals from the blood which may cause cellular damage in many diseases, and may be beneficial with respect to tumors and atherosclerosis. Certain types of skin tumors and ulcer problems in the stomach may be less common with increased catechin intake. Catechins are showing some beneficial effects in HIV, herpes simplex and hepatitis virus infection research.

14

WHAT IS LACTOBACILLUS ACIDOPHILUS?

Lactobacillus acidophilus is a common bacteria found in the intestinal tract of most humans. It is sometimes called the "good bacteria." Lactobacillus acidophilus has been linked to proper digestion and other important activities in the human body. Some recent studies have focused on the nutritional benefits of this particular organism. Lactobacillus acidophilus evidences potential in preventing or controlling intestinal infections, and shows beneficial effects on serum cholesterol levels. Additional beneficial effects relate to carcinogens and cancer formation, and in the improvement of lactose digestion in certain types of patients. (If these people consume milk products containing lactobacillus acidophilus, some currently available evidence indicates that L-acidophilus has an inhibitory action on the bacteria Camphylobacter pylori {associated with some stomach ulcers}. This inhibitory action may be of some future help to patients when Camphylobacter pylori is involved in their stomach ulcer disease.)

Lactobacillus acidophilus is also used to treat herpes simplex (fever blisters) and diarrhea, particularly when the intestinal tract has been significantly depleted of this friendly bacteria, as happens with the consumption of antibiotics.

Animal studies, especially with mice, suggest that treatment with certain types of milk fermented with lactobacillus present seems to have a protective effect on other types of bacterial infections, specifically against salmonella. Human applications of this particular information are still pending. This same bacteria has been studied as a dietary supplement to help lower cholesterol in humans. Animal studies also suggest that milk active with lactobacillus acidophilus can be used as an aid and adjunct against gastrointestinal infections due to other bacteria such as shigella.

Other experiments show that certain strains of acidophilus may be recommended as highly active antagonists for the treatment and prevention of some types of intestinal bacterial problems. Several studies have shown that the presence of lactobacillus acidophilus may have some useful effects on the biliary system or the liver/gall bladder, and the production of cholesterol. Apparently, this results from an action of the bacteria itself which decongregates or breaks up bile salts.

In summary, lactobacillus acidophilus seems to be an important factor in maintaining some regulation of the occurrence of intestinal infections, exerting some beneficial effects on cholesterol levels and lipid metabolism, perhaps having an inhibitory effect on the formation of certain types of cancers, as well as interfering with other bacteria which might cause ulcer disease in the gastrointestinal tract.

15

THE POWER OF GARLIC

Garlic is an herb that was valued as an exchange medium in ancient Egypt and its virtues were described in an inscription on the Cheops pyramid. Garlic has had an important dietary and medicinal role throughout history. The folk uses of garlic have ranged from the treatment of leprosy in humans to managing clotting disorders in horses. During the Middle Ages, physicians prescribed the herb to cure deafness; and Native Americans used garlic as a remedy for earaches, flatulence and scurvy.

We know that garlic contains chemical constituents which have antibiotic, fat-lowering and detoxification effects on the body. Early research indicates that garlic may alter the cancer process. Garlic also has antioxidant properties. These properties affect the levels of fat in the blood. Garlic's antioxidant properties have good effects on the function of platelets (the blood's clotting mechanism cells), on dissolving clots, and on blood pressure. Some believe that the effects of garlic are related to decreasing hardening of the arteries.

Fresh garlic is a source of numerous vitamins, minerals and trace elements, although many are found in only minute quantities. Garlic contains the highest sulfur content of any member of the Allium genus. Two trace elements, germanium and selenium, are found in detectable quantities and have been postulated to play a role in the herb's anti-tumor effect since they improve host immunity and "normalize" the oxygen utilization of neoplastic (tumor) cells.

When the bulb of garlic is ground, the enzyme *allinase* is released. (This results in the conversion of alliin to 2 propenesulfenic acid which dimerzes to form allicin.) Allicin gives the characteristic pungent odor to crushed garlic and is believed to be responsible for some of the pharmacologic activity of the plant.

Researchers at China's Shandong Academy of Medical Science reported the effects of allicin as an antioxidant. Allicin increased the levels of two important antioxidant enzymes in the blood—catalase and glutathione peroxidase. This discovery confirmed the antioxidant and free radical scavenging potential of allicin. Researchers in Japan studied the sulfur compounds in aged garlic extract (a popular deodorized form of garlic) and found five sulfur compounds that inhibited fat peroxidation in the liver, thus preventing a reaction that is considered to be one of the main features of aging in liver cells. According to this research, the sulfur compounds alone appeared to be approximately one thousand times more potent in antioxidant activity than the crude, aged garlic extract itself.

Cholesterol is composed of several different components one of which is the low density lipoprotein fraction (LDL). A study conducted by Tulane University states that total cholesterol levels in those taking garlic tablets dropped by 8% and LDL cholesterol (the "bad" cholesterol) was reduced by 11%.

Garlic administration has been reported to increase fibrinolytic activity. (Fibrinolytic refers to the disintegration or dissolution of *fibrin*, especially by enzymatic activity. Fibrin is the insoluble protein end product of blood coagulation.) Some investigators believe that garlic's ability to reduce cholesterol, triglycerides and LDL, increase HDL, reduce platelet adhesiveness and increase fibrinolytic activity can combine to significantly decrease the risk of atherosclerotic disease.

There is no doubt that garlic has a distinctive taste and smell; and peoples' attitudes toward garlic have a lot to do with its consumption. Some demographic data suggest that the lower-than-normal incidence of atherosclerotic disease among people living in some areas of Spain and Italy may be due, in part, to the routine consumption of garlic in those regions.

A recent study made by researchers at the Clinical Research Center in New Orleans concluded that a garlic preparation of 1.3% allicin, when administered in a large dose, appeared to lower diastolic blood pressure. Although no statistical significance was achieved in systolic blood pressure, a definite trend was observed.

Studies are currently being done on the scavenging effects of garlic components on free radicals in the bloodstream. Most evidence points toward the necessity of further research into the possible role of garlic in the prevention of cancer in humans.

Garlic contains *ajoene*, an extract that definitely inhibits the clumping together of platelets. This action helps prevent plaque buildup in arteries. If taken regularly, garlic is also known to induce a definite decrease of triglycerides (substances in the blood related to vascular disease).

Diallyl sulfide (DAS) is an organosulfur compound that accounts for the flavor and smell associated with garlic and has been shown to inhibit a number of chemically induced forms of cancer. Studies have shown that garlic powder has excellent antioxidant activity and is a good hydroxyl radical scavenger. Hydroxyl radicals are related to many harmful processes in the body.

Garlic may also be useful as a preventive for certain types of embolic and thromboembolic mechanisms. It is well known that garlic and compounds of garlic inhibit the growth of animal tumors and modify the activity of different chemicals that can cause cancer. This is a process whereby garlic actually helps a certain type of cell (called macrophage) in the blood or tissue, and the T-cell (or T-Lymphocyte), which is another immune system cell.

In cardiovascular disease and conditions where clotting is a problem, garlic may be used as a substitute for patients who are sensitive to aspirin. Many patients who take garlic or garlic substitutes show lower total cholesterol, lower triglycerides, and a feeling of "well being."

In summary, garlic has many different beneficial effects on the human body. Garlic shows a great deal of promise as a dietary method of modifying atherosclerosis or hardening of the arteries, blood flow, clotting diseases, relationships to cancer initiation, relationships to cholesterol triglycerides, hypertension, and in providing a sense of "well being." In addition, garlic certainly gives our diet a new flavor!

16

THE PINEAPPLE PLANT AND BROMELAIN

The pineapple plant (Ananas comosus) has been shown to contain at least four distinct cysteine proteases (enzymes). One of these—bromelain—is one of the major proteases in the pineapple fruit. This particular product is absorbed unchanged from the intestinal tract of animals at a rate of about 40% and has several benefits. Bromelain helps in conditions of swelling or edema, has an anti-inflammatory property and an ability to inhibit coagulation or clotting effects in certain types of situations.

Apparently, bromelain helps the activity of serum in the blood, especially with relationship to breaking up fiber and clots, and also in the inhibition of fibrinogen synthesis, which is part of the clotting mechanism. Bromelain also seems to have a direct breakdown effect on fiber and fibrinogen.

Much recent research has concentrated around the prostaglandin synthesis, a system which mediates pain in the body. It is now known that bromelain acts as an anti-prostaglandin type of compound.

In some animal studies, bromelain even inhibits certain types of artificially induced tumors. It seems to have a beneficial effect in some types of skeletal muscle injuries and skeletal muscle damage.

Further interest in this particular compound shows that bromelain affects T-cells (immune cells that fight malignant cells), specifically enhancing T-cell monocyte grouping. The data suggests that members of the bromelain sensitive group of surface molecules may act advantageously as far as the human T-cell activation is concerned.

In summary, both animal and human studies indicate that the cysteine protease bromelain from the pineapple plant has many beneficial effects. Apparently, these effects are related to the immune system, to the T-cells, to anti-inflammatory properties, to cutting down on swelling, to the dissolving of clots, and to interface with undesired aspects of the clotting mechanism. In addition, bromelain shows beneficial effects on the swelling and inflammation associated with soft tissue injuries.

17

INDOLES AND BREAST CANCER

Indoles are complex chemicals which, according to laboratory and animal studies, apparently promote anti-tumor activity. In animals, indoles seem to have beneficial effects in prostatic tumors and various types of breast cancers.

Research studies have demonstrated a strong association between estrogen metabolism and the incidence of breast cancer. Researchers have therefore sought pharmacological means of favorably altering both metabolism and subsequent risk. Indole-3-carbinol, obtained from cruciferous vegetables (e.g., kale, brussels sprouts, cabbage and broccoli), is a known inducer of oxidative (P-450) metabolism in animals. Upon investigation of the effects in humans of short term oral exposure to this indole compound (6–7 mg/kg/day over 7 days), the subjects were given a radiometric test which provided a highly specific and reproducible measure of estrogen (estradiol 2 hydroxylation) before and after exposure to Indole-3-carbinol(I 3 C). In a group of twelve healthy volunteers, the average extent of reduction of cancer risk increased by approximately 50% during this short exposure, affecting men and women equally.

The urinary excretion of two key estrogen metabolites, (2hydroxylation and estriol) was also measured. It was found that the excretion of 2hydroxylation relative to that of estriol was significantly increased by I 3 C (further confirming the ongoing induction of 2hydroxylation).

These results indicate that I 3 C predictably alters endogenous estrogen metabolism toward increased catechol estrogen production, and may thereby provide a novel dietary means for reducing cancer risk.

18

PECTIN

Pectin is found in the cell walls of all plant tissue where it acts as an intercellular "cement" giving the plant rigidity. The compound is found at concentrations of 15% to 30% in the fiber of fruits, vegetables, legumes and nuts. Lemon and orange rinds are among the richest sources of pectin, containing up to 30% of this polysaccharide. Pectin is also found in the roots of most plants.

One of the best effects of pectin supplementation is its ability to lower human blood lipoprotein levels. Most studies have evaluated its ingestion in combination with other gums. For example, a mixture of guar and apple pectin in combination with apple pomaces was evaluated in fifteen diabetic women. Ingestion of the mixture before meals resulted in a significant decrease in total cholesterol levels and triglycerides, although HDL cholesterol levels remained relatively stable.

Dietary fibers have been associated with a reduction in the risk of colon cancer and this may also apply to pectin. The possible direct mechanisms include the binding of carcinogens to undergraded dietary fibers, and the absorption of water by these fibers to increase stool bulk and shorten gastrointestinal transit time.

Pectin has also been investigated for its ability to reduce the consequences of exposure to radiation. Persons exposed to radiation after the Chernobyl accident were given pectin supplements. These had a beneficial effect on the antioxidant level of the hematologic systems, and helped normalize their triglyceride and albumin levels. Pectin supplements appear to act as "enteroabsorbents," protecting against the accumulation of ingested radioactivity.

In summary, pectin is a natural polysaccharide that forms thick colloidal solutions in water. It is added to processed foods to create texture. Medicinally, the compound has been widely used in antidiarrheal products, serving as a stool-forming agent. It also appears to lower blood lipoprotein levels. Pectin is generally well tolerated although it may interfere with the absorption of dietary nutrients.

19

THE NEED FOR FRUITS AND VEGETABLES

The need for fruits and vegetables in the human diet has been studied extensively for many years. The importance of certain vegetables has even been mentioned in the Bible, in the Prophecy of Daniel (chapter 1, verses 8–16). Modern scientific research and studies throughout the world over the past ten years have emphasized the value of a diet which is high in fruit and vegetable intake. Many of these studies are currently ongoing and others have already been completed. In summary, these studies show specific benefits of fruits and vegetables to humans. When fruits and vegetables are consumed in high quantities, we are placed at a lower risk for heart disease, cancer and many chronic and acute disorders.

The components of fruits and vegetables which seem to offer the greatest benefits appear to be fiber, food enzymes, antioxidants, trace minerals and food actives. There are specific diseases and disorders which seem to be beneficially altered, prevented, or modified by particular fruits and vegetables.

The medical literature from many countries such as the United States, Russia, China, Canada, Argentina, Australia, Italy, Japan and Sweden is replete with studies which show the significant reduction in risk of cancer, heart disease and chronic diseases associated with the high consumption of both fruits and vegetables. In all situations, a higher intake of vegetables and fruits has placed most patients at a lower risk for diverse types of cancers, probably through different biomedical mechanisms.

Research Around The World

Italian studies show that there is a consistent pattern of protection for all epithelial cancers (specifically in the esophagus, stomach and GI tract) for those who have a high vegetable intake. If fruit intake is high, there is a protective effect for cancer of the upper digestive tract and respiratory tract also. Fruits and vegetables also seem to have some protective effect on the urinary tract neoplasm rate. Low intake of vegetables, fruits and carotenoids is consistently associated with an increased risk of lung cancer in both prospective and retrospective studies.

A study in China showed that male tin miners who had a reduced dietary intake of yellow and light green vegetables had a significant increase in lung cancer. Reduced intake of tomatoes correlated with a statistically significant increase of lung cancer. In other words, intake of fruits and vegetables and tomatoes was helpful in decreasing cancer risk.

In the United States, a study from the Department of Pathology at Louisiana State University Medical Center in New Orleans reported that dietary studies have been consistent in finding an approximate 50% reduction in the risk of lung cancer associated with a high consumption of carotene-containing fruits and vegetables. Clinical trials are presently being done to try to analyze the significant factors which offer the best protection and the important particulates of fruits and vegetables which offer the protection in groups such as heavy smokers, miners and asbestos workers.

The National Cancer Institute has done a study which shows a relationship between dietary intake of fruits and vegetables (especially if they are fresh) and the risk of oral or mouth cancer among blacks. The results seem to indicate that there is a protective effect in both men and women, although it was slightly stronger for men. (Researchers believe that the consumption of nitrate-containing meats was linked to an increased risk among men and felt that the lower consumption of fruits among blacks in this particular study might have some contributory effect to the fact that they had higher rates of mouth and pharyngeal cancer.)

Studies in Australia regarding the risk of colon cancer have shown that those who had a high intake of vegetables and fruit, especially females who had a greater intake of onions and legumes, were at decreased risk. For males, those who had a greater intake of green leafy vegetables and carrots and cabbage had a lower risk. These studies also show that those who have a low fiber, low vegetable intake and a high intake of beef and beer, have a higher incidence of polyps of the colon or colon rectal polyps.

Diet and cancer of the colon and rectum were studied in a case-controlled study in China. Again, green vegetables seemed to have a strong protective effect against colon rectal cancer. Excess alcohol intake was found to be an important risk factor also for developing colon cancer and male rectal cancer.

In Argentina, studies have reported that the intake of vegetables is associated with a statistically significant decrease in the risk for colon cancer.

Across the Board

In a review article, a statistically significant protective effect of fruit and vegetable consumption was found in 128 of 156 dietary studies. For most cancer sites, persons with low fruit and vegetable intake experience about twice the risk of cancer compared to those with a high intake of fruits and vegetables. Fruits, in particular, seem significantly protective for cancer of the esophagus, the mouth and the larynx (or voice box). Strong evidence of the protective effect of fruit and vegetable consumption was seen also in cancers of the pancreas and stomach as well as in colon rectal and urinary bladder cancer.

Today, many of the major medical schools are teaching young physicians the importance of fruits and vegetables in the diet and the relationship between the dietary consumption of a nutritious diet and the development of cancer, heart disease and chronic disease.

The Need for Education

There are many difficulties in actually consuming fruits and vegetables in the quantity, volume and variety that has been recommended by major health organizations throughout this country and throughout the world. Cost, availability, storage and taste are all important factors.

Education remains critical in the alteration of the human diet and nutritional status as it exists today in this world. Surveys have shown extreme discrepancies between recommended dietary guidelines and actual dietary consumption. These have enhanced the need for educational solutions. In one survey on a particular day, 45% of respondents had no fruits or vegetables, 27% had three or more servings of vegetables and only 29% had two or more servings of fruits. Only 9% had consumed recommended amounts. The choice of vegetables lacked variety and the fiber intake was only about 17 grams, which is below recommended amounts.

The National Cancer Institute, the American Cancer Society and many other health organizations throughout this country are currently conducting a twenty-five million dollar advertising campaign to try to encourage you to modify your diet to include five servings of raw, fresh fruits and vegetables every day. The effects of this campaign are clearly visible already. If you shop in some of the larger grocery stores or supermarkets in just about any major city you will see the slogan, "5 servings a day of fresh fruits and vegetables recommended by the National Cancer Institute," actually stamped on the plastic bags that you put your fruits and vegetables in when you purchase them. These agencies also would advise you to decrease your cigarette smoking, decrease fat intake, cut back on alcohol consumption, cut back on salt intake and modify the way you prepare your food.

Health Producing Components of Fruits and Vegetables

Fiber
The first component of fruits and vegetables which offers numerous protective benefits to us is fiber. Plant fiber is an important factor in the human diet. An increased risk of cancer has been noted in those diets that were high in protein intake or fat intake and not in those with high cellulose (fiber) intake. The usual high fat, low fiber diet of the Western world is related to the risk of cancer of the colon, pancreas, breast, prostate, ovary and endometrium. The majority of studies at many cancer centers throughout the world have shown a protective effect associated with fiber rich diets.

Foods which ferment in the colon are associated with less colon rectal cancer. Canadian studies have shown that vegetable fiber, specifically broccoli, cabbage and carrots are more effective in stimulating fermentation in the colon. Vegetable fiber is superior to the traditional dietary fiber from corn, rice and wheat consumed in the Western world.

Fiber is extremely beneficial in the diet insofar as it absorbs harmful compounds in the intestinal tract which increase the risk of certain types of cancer and pre-cancerous states.

Enzymes

The protective and preventive effects of enzymes have been well documented in Chapter 1. Enzymes which are active in raw unprocessed vegetables and fruits have a detoxifying or inactivating effect on certain harmful chemicals which tend to cause cancer in humans. These very enzymes also inhibit, block or decrease the ability of other cancer-causing compounds to bind to or interfere with cellular DNA. By these mechanisms, enzymes offer protective effects for the cells and prevent cancer development. Cruciferous vegetables, specifically those of the genus brassica (which includes broccoli), contain components which induce, produce and activate other enzymes in the body's metabolism which decrease the risk of cancer.

Antioxidants

Raw uncooked fruits and vegetables are a main source of our dietary antioxidants. These include vitamins C, E and beta carotene. All of these have a critical place in the prevention of cancer by their antioxidant activity. Current research indicates a tremendously important association between the antioxidants and the intake of fruits and vegetables in the human system. Dietary supplementation with a specific antioxidant such as vitamin C, vitamin E, beta-carotene or vitamin A may offer some benefits, but most authorities still recommend obtaining these products from natural sources such as fruits and vegetables if at all possible.

Antioxidant carotenoids which are common in fruits and vegetables may be grouped or characterized predominately as beta-carotene, alpha-carotene, lutein and lycopenes and cryptoxanthin. The major food which contains alpha-carotene is carrots. Carrots and broccoli are a main source of beta-carotene. Orange juices and blends of orange juice are rich in cryptoxanthin. Tomatoes and tomato products are important sources of lycopenes. Lutein is found in spinach and broccoli. Increased intake of carotenoid rich fruits and vegetables is associated with reduced risk of lung cancer.

Another antioxidant which is present in moderate to high amounts in fresh fruits and vegetables is glutathione. Most forms of cooking and preparing food appear to decrease the glutathione content. Canned and other processed food contains substantially less glutathione than fresh fruits and vegetables. Dietary intake of glutathione may be an important factor in the resistance to cancer.

Another antioxidant called *flavonoid* is found in many fruits and vegetables (such as apples and onions) and red wine. (Green tea is a rich source of flavonoids also.) Flavonoid intake seems to cut down the death rate from heart disease significantly. Also, it has shown cancer-preventive activity in lab animals.

Lycopene is important because it contributes to the antioxidation defense system of the human. Increasing your dietary intake of antioxidants from plants such as fruits and vegetables not only will decrease your risk of cancer but will also help fight many diseases such as the common cold, diabetes, Alzheimer's disease and heart disease. This is true because the antioxidant vitamins C, E, and beta-carotene counter the damaging effects of free radicals which constitute the main cause of a wide variety of disease processes in the body.

The National Academy of Sciences in its dietary guideline recommendations of 1991 stated that some fruits and vegetables should be consumed in their fresh raw state since some vitamin C (one of the more important antioxidants) is lost even in brief careful cooking.

Green and yellow vegetables such as carrots, broccoli, winter squash, spinach, kale and collard greens provide rich sources of beta-carotene. Citrus fruits including oranges, tangerines and grapefruit are known to be excellent sources of the antioxidant vitamin C.

Women with a lower intake of vitamins C, E and other antioxidants have an increased risk for cervical dysplasia or certain types of pre-cancerous lesions. Also, vitamin C is reported to have beneficial effects in diabetics in decreasing the amount of glucose that is bound to certain proteins in the blood; and evidence suggests this process may be beneficial for diabetics in the long-term.

Vitamin C also has an antihistamine effect, and as such should be consumed adequately by people who have allergy problems. Many patients with a common cold have felt for years that an increase in their intake of their vitamin C seemed to ameliorate or modify their cold. Recent research confirms that increasing your intake of vitamin C will modify the length and severity of a cold.

Vitamin E supplementation has been associated with a reduced risk of oral cancer in a study done by the National Cancer Institute. In addition, many studies have shown that vitamin E has beneficial effects related to heart disease, angina and low density lipoproteins.

Trace Minerals

The importance of fruits and vegetables as sources of trace minerals such as zinc, magnesium, chromium, selenium and copper cannot be emphasized enough. These are all critical to many enzyme systems and interrelate to each other in cellular functions. Zinc, selenium and copper are especially important in the retina's metabolism. Chromium relates to energy production and the ability to mobilize fat. Deficiencies of magnesium may lead to problems with blood pressure, diabetes and asthma. Sources of traces minerals include such foods as dried fruits for chromium, grains for zinc and leafy green vegetables such as spinach and broccoli for magnesium.

Food Actives

Food actives include the Isothiocyanates found in broccoli, cabbage and cauliflower, the Monoterpenes found in citrus fruits, the Organosulfer compounds found in garlic and cruciferous vegetables and the Glucobrassicin, Polyphenols and Indoles found in broccoli and other cruciferous vegetables. They are important in counteracting the effects of cancer and heart disease.

Indoles are very complex chemicals, but their beneficial effects (both in studies in the lab and actual animal studies) relate to anti-tumor growth or activity. Animal studies seem to indicate beneficial effects on prostatic tumors, various types of breast cancers and colon cancer. Indoles appear to activate some enzymes which break down the female hormone estrogen. This seems helpful in reducing breast cancer. Indoles are found in several fruits and vegetables in their raw uncooked state.

Polyphenols are being studied as far as their ability to shield sensitive structures in the body from carcinogens and to stimulate the repair of DNA and cells which have been damaged by carcinogens. Also, cell membranes have been strengthened or stabilized by polyphenols.

Another food active is natural D-glucaric acid which is found in broccoli, cabbage, bean sprouts, cherries, apples and oranges. Animal studies show it helps lower LDL cholesterol and suppress cell growth which may lead to breast and colon cancer. Sulforaphane found in broccoli and related vegetables increases the production of an enzyme which neutralizes certain carcinogens before they cause damage.

Licorice derivatives from legumes (certain vegetables) contain triterpenoids which appear to slow cancer cell growth or return cell growth to normal.

Thus there are many methods by which the active components of fruits and vegetables seem to produce their protective effect in the cancer process and many studies are currently underway.

The Challenge of Getting It Five Times a Day

It takes a tremendous amount of energy and time to obtain fruits and vegetables in this fast-paced world. They must be purchased when they are available, if they can be found, and they must be consumed when fresh or the beneficial effects seem to be decreased. The money that must be spent to purchase what the National Cancer Institute and American Cancer Society suggest, which is about five servings per day of raw uncooked fruits and vegetables, is no small amount. In one particular instance an individual shopped at a local food store which had low prices and it was found that it took approximately forty-five minutes to select out five fruits and five vegetables to provide some variety to the diet. The cost of those particular fruits and vegetables was approximately $10.00. It is reasonable to say that an average person would have to spend a tremendous amount of time and several thousand dollars per person per year to try to obtain five servings of raw fruits and vegetables (if they could be even found). The fact that consumers are not interested in consuming raw fruits and vegetables is no small wonder due to the expense, the time involved and the waste that occurs in trying to store such compounds.

In spite of the encouragement to increase our intake of fruits, it has been shown (at least in certain populations) that those who did consume high amounts of fruits over a long period of time had a higher association of dental cavities related to the sugar content of the fruits. Thus, one is faced with the problem of an increased risk for dental caries with high fruit consumption. At the same time it is now well known that fruits are an essential protective agent against several forms of carcinoma. The dilemma here is to try to find some method whereby one could consume fruits and vegetables, specifically fruits, without increasing the risk of dental caries and thus creating another problem. It was found that the consumption of a high amount of apples, and to a lesser degree grapes, contributed significantly to dental caries although it seemed to have a beneficial effect on the amount of periodontal status. It was also reported in another study that the enamel of the tooth seems to erode more quickly when a person was exposed to fruit juice or juices as marketed. The erosion effect was about five to eight times higher in juice consumption than in eating the fruit in its natural state. It would certainly be advantageous to determine a method of obtaining fruits in a form that allowed their consumption without increasing the risk of dental cavities.

Summary

If you're not getting fruits and vegetables five times a day, every day, we understand why. In reading this book, however, you should understand why it is important to try. If you can't always "get it five times a day" but have other alternatives, add those to your lifestyle and habits. Teach your children to do the same.

For Further Reading

BOOKS

Attwood, Charles, M.D. *Dr. Attwood's Low-Fat Prescription for Kids*. New York: Penguin, 1995.

Crackower, Sydney, H.B., M.D. *Creating Your Own Good Health*. New Vision Publications.

Dorian, Terry, Ph.D. *Health Begins in Him*. Lafayette, LA: Huntington House, 1995.

Haas, Elson M., M.D. *Staying Healthy with Nutrition*. Berkeley, CA: Celestial Arts, 1992.

Howell, Dr. Edward. *Enzyme Nutrition*. Garden City Park, N.Y.: Avery Publishing Group, 1985.

Jensen, Dr. Bernard. *Foods That Heal*, Garden City Park, N.Y.: Avery Publishing Group, 1993.

Mindell, Earl. *Vitamin Bible*. New York: Warner Books, 1991.

Santillo, Humbart. *Food Enzymes—The Missing Link to Radiant Health*. Second Edition, Prescott, AZ: Hohm Press, 1993.

Santillo, Humbart. *The Basics of Intuitive Eating*. Prescott, AZ: Hohm Press, 1994.

Shila M.E., Young, V.R. *Modern Nutrition in Health and Disease*. 7th ed., Philadelphia: Lea and Febiger, 1988.

Walker, Norman W., D.Sc., Ph.D., *Colon Health*. Prescott, AZ: Norwalk Press, 1995.

JOURNALS

Block, G., et al. "Fruit, Vegetables and Cancer Prevention: A Review of the Epidemiological Evidence." *Nutr Cancer* 18 (1): I-29 (1992)

Bruce, R.A. "Nutritional Compliance and Macular Degeneration Symposium." *Oc Surg News* 1991; April (Suppl): 11–12.9

"Eye Disease Case-Control Study Group, Antioxidant Status and Neovascular Age-Related Macular Degeneration." *Arch Ophthamol* 111:104–109 (Jan 1993)

"Eye Disease Case-Control Study Group, Risk factors for Neovascular Age-Related Macular Degeneration." *Arch Ophthamol* 110:1701–8 (1992)

Gridley, G., et al. "Vitamins Supplement Use and Reduced Risk of Oral and Pharyngeal Cancer." *AMJ Epidemiology* 135(10): 1083–1092 (15 May 1992)

Johnson, K., Kligman, E.W., "Preventative Nutrition: An 'optimal' diet for older adults." *Geriatrics* 1992; 47(10): 56–60

Pitts, G.D. "Ultraviolet Absorbing Spectacle Lenses, Contact Lenses, and Intraocular Lenses." *Optom & Vis Sci* 1990; 67:430–40

Rimms, E.B., et al. "Vitamin E Supplementation and Risk of Coronary Heart Disease Among Men." *Circulation* 86: I-436 (Oct 1992)

I AM INTERESTED IN:

1. ☐ More information from (choose only one name)

   a. ☐ Dr. Bohn
   b. ☐ Dr. Crackower
   c. ☐ Rodney Langlinais
      on (your question) _____

      _____

      _____

2. ☐ Any information on a home-based business involving neutraceutical products.

My Name _____

Address _____

City _____ State _____ Zip _____

Phone (____) _____ Best time to call: _____

Must be completed for us to respond. Thank you.

COMMENTS ON BOOK:

_____

_____

_____

_____

_____

Your signature below allows I.M.M. to use your testimony in future promotions.

_____   _____
SIGNATURE   DATE

_____   _____
OCCUPATION   TITLE

**Intercontinental Marketing
and Management**

P.O. Box 31772

Lafayette, Louisiana 70593-1772

ATTENTION: Public Relations Department